Nutrition for Life

Food & Fitness Tips for Success

By Joyce Ainsworth

2014 ©Copyright Joyce Ainsworth.
1st Edition

Printed in the U.S.A.

ISBN – 13: 978-1505502497
ISBN – 10: 150 5502497

Cover by Joyce Ainsworth

Acknowledgments

I am grateful for the love and support of my friends and staff at my home church Crossgates Baptist Church. They have been willing to step out in faith and provide support for the ministry of First Place 4 Health (FP4H). Thank you for allowing my ministry to flourish and grow here in this place!

I am also very thankful for all the friends and members who have come through my classes. You have touched my life in so many special ways and as we have studied, prayed, and grown together, my desire is that you have been inspired to find real life change. You have encouraged me in so many ways through the years. Thank you for pushing me to be the best I can be for Jesus.

I will be forever grateful to the staff of First Place 4 Health. Their willingness to follow the Lord's calling through the ministry of FP4H has radically changed my life.

I am grateful to Jan Duke, June Chapko and my husband Glenn for their invaluable work of editing this project. A great big "Thank You" for going above and beyond to make this project the best it could be.

I want to especially take a moment just to mention and personally thank Donna Conerly for her invaluable help with the nutrition information in this book. Donna and I studied together many long hours to become certified as specialist in fitness nutrition. The day we received our certificates from International Sports Sciences Association (ISSA) was a day of celebration! Donna and I knew this certification would allow us to help many to take their food and fitness to a new level. With Donna's invaluable help and by the Lord's direction these food and fitness tips will help everyone take the next step to success. It is an honor to work alongside dear ones like Donna who love the Lord and allow that to be reflected in their work. May the Lord receive all the Glory!

Dedication

"Call to me and I will answer you, and I will tell you great and mighty things, which you do not know" (Jeremiah 33:3 NASB).

This Nutrition for Life book is lovingly and affectionately dedicated to my Savior and Friend Jesus
He has truly made real and lasting life change possible.

~~All for His Glory~~

To my beloved husband Glenn who has always loved "both" of me! Words are inadequate to express my love and gratitude for your steadfast love, encouragement, and support through this life-change journey! Thank you for being willing to run the race.

To my children Heather, David, Daniel, Jason, and Brad
My prayer is for each of you to find real life change through the power of Christ!

To all my readers

Change Your Mind! Change Your Body! Change Your Life!

Table of Contents

Introduction

Health Matters!

How many times have we lost weight simply to regain that weight plus some more? Most of us know "how" to lose weight but few know how to lose the weight and keep it off forever.....I am a regular girl who by the grace of the Lord I have achieved a remarkable weight loss of 192 pounds; but the real success has been in developing a plan to maintain my new lifestyle that is simple, practical and easy enough for anyone to follow.

Throughout the pages of this book I will share some personal strategies with you along with tips on food, exercise, my 12 super foods, some of my favorite go to websites, menu planning, grocery shopping, healthy substitutions and other health related subjects that will help you build your own strategy for being successful at real and lasting "Life Change". I will challenge you to change your mind and love your body.

The desire is to bring encouragement to you to seek and develop a solid plan that will be simple, practical and easy to follow so that you can be equipped to develop a healthy new lifestyle that really works for you. In this fast pace life finding balance in midst of a busy life can truly be life changing.
Don't wait another day to start getting healthy! Good health really does matter.

It really is time to:
Change Your Mind ~ Change Your Body ~ Change Your Life ~

Faithfully His
Joyce

Walking with God:

O God, You are my God,
Earnestly I seek you; my soul thirsts for you
My body longs for you, in a dry and weary land
Where there is no water,
I have seen you in the sanctuary and beheld your power and your glory
Because your love is better than life, my lips will glorify you!
I will praise you as long as I live, and in your name I will lift up my hands
My soul will be satisfied as with the richest of foods
With singing lips my mouth will praise you
Psalm 63: 1-5

It is truly amazing to me as we "Grow in Christ" how much the real meaning behind this statement changes. As a young Christian I thought walking with God meant showing up for church on Sunday and Wednesday, trying to do the right things, raising my children to do the same, being an example that others could follow, and having great ideas that would minister to others and help them grow.

All great and noble ideals or so I thought at the time; all along I was truly expecting God to bless "my" ideas, "my" ministry.

As God has taken me through my own personal journey I am reminded of a statement in the scripture, Ephesians 4:22-24, where it talks about putting off the old self and putting on the new self. Why? Because we were created to be in a relationship with God and as we walk down this road of relationship with God we will become more like God. Not God but like God. As we walk with Him we begin to be a reflection of Him. We will take on His mind, His thoughts will be our thoughts and His character will become our character.

The hardest thing for most of us to comprehend is the fact that God longs to help us. He is eager for a real, personal, and authentic relationship with each of us. He does not want to be a part of my life and your life but he wants to be woven into the fabric of our lives in such a way that He becomes our life.

As all things in my life have been I find this has been and I believe will continue to be a process, a journey. Most of us want "instant results" but real life change is a decision we choose to make. It is a decision we will have to make every day. Same is true with our relationship with God. Walking with God does not happen by accident or from just being in the room. It is a clear, conscience, decision; it is truly a process, a daily journey.

In Psalm 62:5 the psalmist says I can find rest for my soul in God alone, that my hope comes from Him. For me to be able to rest in this truth I must "do" several things. I must stay tuned into God. I do that through the renewing of my mind, I spend time in His word daily, I listen for His voice, I pray and call on His strength because "His" strength is sufficient and mine is not. I must "put off" not cover up but put off my old ways, habits and hang ups and "put on" the Mind of Christ. I believe the only way we can do that is to "walk" with God daily in prayer, Bible study, and become a "seeker" for His direction, I look for where He is working and then join Him in that place.

I have to be willing to be changed by the touch of the Savior! Walking with God is and will continue to be a journey for me and through this I find that I can wait patiently for Him to work all things; even the troubles, for my ultimate good because He is my enduring hope. He is truly the lover of my soul! Walking with God allows me to find His presence, provision and protection. God alone truly satisfies fully. I find my joy in worshiping You, My Lord!

Oh God You are my God, earnestly I seek You. You are my LIFE!

Faithfully His
Joyce

Nutrition for Life

Food & Fitness Tips for Success

By Joyce Ainsworth

Chapter 1 ~ Nutrition for "LIFE" Plan

Food is very important to all of us and learning to make good healthy food choices does not make us weird or different. I used to live to eat and now I have learned to eat to live. Eating with a purpose is a "learned" behavior and it was a process that started in my mind. I call this my "Nutrition for Life Plan"

I base this plan on the following scripture:

All things are lawful for me, but not all things are profitable. All things are lawful for me, but I will not be mastered by anything.
1 Corinthians 6:12

Or, Do you not know that your body is a temple of the Holy Spirit who is in you, whom you have received from God, and that you are not your own?
For you have been bought with a price: therefore glorify God in your body
1 Corinthians 6: 19 & 20

Suggested Changes:

➢ Commit to a weekly goal of some sort: _____
Setting a goal helps you better plan for your week. This goal can be focused on exercise and/or food. I set a food and exercise goal. They should go hand in hand and work together for your success.

➢ Determine Your Calorie Range: calories per day (FP4H Members Guide Page 120) or you can also visit the following website: **http://caloriecount.about.com/** Your calorie range is needed info for you to be able to track your food daily.

➢ Variety in nutrient packed fruits and veggies is the "Key" to unlocking the door to your body's highest potential. Your body will perform better when you feed it the right fuel. Variety keeps us from getting bored and burned out on the same foods. Variety is the spice of life so keep your plan interesting.

➤ Recommended Daily Amount of Food from each Group per day (FP4H Members Guide Page 123) this will be based on your calorie range that is right for your age and activity level.

FRUIT~ (_____ cups) VEGGIES~ (___ to _____ cups) GRAINS~ (_____ oz)
MILK (Dairy) ~ (___ cups) MEAT&BEANS~ (_____ oz) on exercise days do _____oz of meat and HEALTHY OILS~ (_____tsp.)

Please note: on the oils this is <u>teaspoons</u> not tablespoons (Review info on healthy oils & how they count in the FP4H Members Guide on pages 146 – 148. Additional and important info can be found in the Simple Ideas for Healthy Living book page 118 thru 126. (It is worth the read)

If you do not have a copy of these books they can be purchased on the First Place 4 Health website at **www.firstplace4health.com**

➤ Add the following vegetables to your plan if you are **not** already eating them Turnip Greens/ Collard Greens/ Green Beans fresh or frozen / Black Beans dried or canned but if you purchase the canned ones; look for the lower sodium varieties/ Cauliflower (raw or steamed)/ Broccoli (raw or steamed)/ Carrots (raw or cooked)/ Squash and Zucchini/ Sweet Potatoes/ Spinach and Mixed Greens/ Romaine/ Leaf Lettuce/ Mushrooms/ Bell Peppers (all colors)/ Tomatoes/ Onions/ Celery/ Brussels Sprouts/ Steamed Cabbage/ Kale/ and last but not least Asparagus.

All these vegetables are really good for you and needed to be added to your plan. Avoid iceberg lettuce because it has no nutritional value for your body.

➤ Add the following fruits to your plan if you are **not** already eating them:
Avocados/ Mangos/ Apples (all varieties)/ Pears/ Peaches/ Plums/ Raspberries/ Blueberries/ Blackberries/ Strawberries/ Kiwi Fruit/ Pomegranates and Pineapple are all great fruit choices and need to be part of your food plan. You can also add watermelon, honeydew and cantaloupe when they are in season.

Oranges, bananas and grapes are higher in natural sugar so try limiting these choices to once a week instead of on an everyday basis.

Always choose fresh or frozen fruit when possible, they are the best choice.

The Skinny on Snacks

If you choose the right snacks they can be good and healthy. Snacks can help you stay on track with your new lifestyle and stay satisfied. Snacks that contain a good mix of protein, carbohydrates, calcium or antioxidants keep your body at its best. Focus on finding snacks that will help fend off a craving without a lot of added fat, sugar or calories. No matter what you choose try to choose well! Making good food choices will make a difference especially in this area. When you need a snack learn to ask yourself; is this a "Quality" food.

You will find additional info on choosing snacks later within this resource.

The Truth about Tracking Your Food

First Place 4 Health has always taught that tracking and keeping a food diary is so important. Whether you want to lose weight or just maintain a healthy lifestyle tracking needs to become a part of your plan. Tracking helps all of us be consistent and consistency brings quicker results. Tracking makes us "think" about what we are really eating, helps us formulate realistic goals, and helps us see our trouble spots like whether we are eating from all the food groups and whether we are eating too few or too many calories. Food tracking also helps us detect whether our plan is in proper balance. Proper balance simply means: Quality, Variety and Quantity. We want to learn to eat a variety of foods in proper quantity and we want them all to be quality foods.

➤ Some helpful websites I use for tracking food are:
Myfitnesspal.com, Spark people, and fit bit, are just a few and I am sure there are other websites and apps out there that can help you be successful. If you e-mail me at **glenna@netdoor.com** I will be happy to send you a copy of several paper trackers that I have used throughout the years.
Any of these methods of tracking will work. Tracking helps you see and find the balance you need in your food plan.
The key to being successful is to "DO IT" consistently

My Nutrition Plan Changes:

Here is your opportunity to begin to build your plan. Write down some of your thoughts and changes you intend to make here.

What is my new goal:

_____

_____

What is my calorie range?

_____

_____

What do my recommended daily food allowances look like for my calorie range:
FRUIT~ (_____ cups) VEGGIES~ (___ to _____ cups)   GRAINS~ (_____ oz)
MILK (Dairy) ~ (___ cups) MEAT&BEANS~ (_____ oz) on exercise days do _____oz of meat and HEALTHY OILS~ (_____tsp.)

What fruits do intend to add to my new plan:

_____

_____

What vegetables do I intend to add to my new plan:

_____

_____

What snacks do I need to add?

_____

_____

What snacks have I been eating that I need to commit not to eat for a while?

_____

_____

Chapter 2 ~ Food is Fuel

Do we really think about food being fuel? Food is the fuel that runs our bodies. The human body is a finely-tuned biological machine, capable of incredible feats of strength, intelligence, memory, learning, and the list goes on. Like any finely-tuned machine, healthy and constant fuel—in our case, food, in the form of protein, carbohydrates, good fats, vitamins and minerals—needs to be readily available and ingested. If not, this machine will slow down, perform poorly and ultimately, stop running

In this chapter I cover some of my foods. These are foods I eat and use on a regular basis. These are some healthy choices you may want to consider adding to your plan as well. These food items are high quality foods with a high nutrient base. Remember food is fuel for your workouts and your everyday life. We need to eat right to stay strong and healthy.
Pray about making the change first then take baby steps to change!

~ Butter ~ Smart Balance buttery spread light with flaxseed oil

**~ Dannon Greek (light and fit) yogurt   80 Calories for a 5.3 oz cup
(Many flavors to choose from try a variety)**

~Tofu Shirataki (angel hair shaped noodles) by House Foods you will find them in the dairy section in most grocery stores. Great option instead of pasta

~ Joseph Pita Bread ~ Flax, Oat Bran and Whole Wheat bread (this is a whole grain food) and a very healthy choice instead of bread.

~ Skinny Girl Stevia ~ comes in a liquid (the only sweetener I use any more) Stevia is from a plant and has replaced all sugar in my home.

~ Philadelphia (1/3 less fat) garden vegetable cream cheese spread (Is great on pizza) and is great for making dips and sauces too!

~<u>The laughing Cow</u>~ Light 50% less fat spreadable cheese wedges (great snack) You can have a wedge of laughing cow and an apple to make a perfect afternoon snack or post workout snack.

~<u>Suzie's Whole Grain</u> brown rice cakes (these are sodium, cholesterol, gluten, Fat and sugar free) I buy these on Amazon. You can find them at most Whole Foods stores as well. These are great with a teaspoon of peanut butter and a sliced strawberry on top; makes a great bedtime snack or dessert.

~ <u>Peanut Butter</u> ~ All natural (check the label) I love to go to the Whole Foods store or fresh market and just make it myself. The fresher it is the better it is.

~<u>Almond Butter</u> ~ All natural (check the label) Almond butter is usually lower in saturated fat than peanut butter. I now go to the Whole Foods store and make my peanut butter and almond butter fresh and on sight. It is better for you and no additives and in truth the cost is about the same as the store bought varieties.

~<u>Uncle Sam Cereal</u>, Toasted Whole Wheat Berry Flakes and Flaxseed Original variety is the one I buy; it comes in a 10 oz box and also a 13oz box depending on the brand you buy. I can get it at Kroger, Wal-Mart and most health food stores. Uncle Sam Cereal is available from U.S. Mills and also Attune Foods.

~ <u>Almond Breeze</u> ~ Unsweetened Chocolate almond milk is only 45 calories a serving and is loaded with calcium. I also buy the almond and coconut blend. It is great for smoothies.

~<u>PB2 – Powdered Peanut Butter</u>: Is great for smoothies and has less fat and sugar than regular peanut butter. It is available in most grocers and online.

~<u>Amazing Grass Green Super food</u>: Great to add to smoothies. It is made with organic green foods. I usually order it on-line from Amazon. SometimesI can find it at GNC but it is much cheaper on-line.

~Happy Puffs Organic Super foods: This is great snack item. I started buying them for my grandbabies and have found that I love them! You can use as a snack or add to yogurt for a little crunch without a lot of fat or calories. It is also a great snack if you are a diabetic because they are very low in carbohydrates. The next time you are in the grocery store check out the baby food isle. You may find a new healthy snack!

~Walden Farms: Most of the Walden farm items are calorie free, sugar free, and fat free. They carry a line of salad dressings, syrups and barbeque sauce. They can be found in most groceries including Wal-Mart.

~ Seeds of Change: Have a variety of rice and other grains. One of our favorites is a Spanish rice with Quinoa, red pepper and corn. It comes in a pouch and is ready in 90 seconds in the microwave. It makes a great healthy choice for single people or individuals that don't have time to do much cooking. For me it is just so convenient and helps me get lunch or dinner on the table quickly.

~Uncle Ben's also carries a line of brown rice products now that are ready in minutes. They also come in single serving and smaller portion packaging. Check out your local grocery to see which ones they carry.

~KIND Bars: Lots of varieties: They make simple all natural products and deliver a healthy snack made only with ingredients you can see and pronounce. This bar is just about all I eat now for a snack.

~Quest Bars: Lots of variety and have a high standard of quality ingredients and protein. These are great when you are working out and need a good balance of protein and carbohydrates. This is my go to work out bar. I order on-line but you can find these at many fitness centers and GNC stores.

~FIT Popcorn: Comes already popped and is about 30 calories a cup. I usually pick this up at Sam's Club or Kroger. It now comes in a variety of flavors.

~Skinny Pop Popcorn: It is also already popped and contains about 39 calories a cup. It is all natural. This is a quality snack food without a bunch of extra stuff. I keep some of this on hand for parties and when my grand kids come over.

Let me finish "My Foods" list with this thought: This list is <u>ever changing</u> and I am constantly adding to and taking away from this list. The more I learn about food the more I try to eat all natural, healthy foods with quality ingredients. I avoid processed foods as much as possible. Remember this is a journey and you cannot make all the changes that need to be made overnight. Start somewhere and make small baby-steps to change. If you mess up then start over and keep practicing until you get it right. Just be willing not to give up. If you keep trying you will be successful.

The Lord will lead you as you go if you are willing to ask. "Life Change" is a process not a onetime event. I am still in a constant state of change. Learn to be a "Food Detective" and seek out all the healthy choices you can make. That mindset and a renewed commitment to a healthy lifestyle will help you learn to enjoy the journey to good health and good food!

My Nutrition Plan Changes:

Write down some of your thoughts and the changes you intend to make here.

_____
_____
_____
_____

What are some new "foods" that I intend to add to my nutrition plan:

_____
_____
_____
_____
_____

Chapter 3 ~ Additional Information & Tips about Food Finds

There isn't a day that goes by when I am not asked what is the best olive oil to use or which is the best peanut butter to buy or which skillet would be the best for sautéing onions and greens. As a Certified Specialist in Fitness Nutrition, cookbook author and blessed big loser, I get asked all sorts of questions everyday about food, fitness and nutrition. I consider it a personal responsibility to be on the lookout for products, cooking tips and fabulous food finds that will enhance my new lifestyle and along the way I love sharing these with each of you.

The following are a few of those Tips and Food Finds:

~Puddings and Jello should be the sugar-free and fat-free varieties if at all possible. Most of us consume way to much sugar and fat in our food plans.

~Peanut butter nabs or crackers If these are part of your food plan then look for the low fat varieties. Most manufactures now carry one that has 25% less fat and may be a healthy way for you to cut back on saturated fat intake.

~Cheese sticks are a great snack food but look for the 2% or low fat varieties. If you buy the ones that are a blend of different cheeses it gives the lower fat varieties more flavor.

~Replace fried foods with steamed, grilled or baked (really work toward this) Fried foods have "No Nutritional Value" for the body. Even veggies when fried become an unhealthy option if you are trying to lose weight and become healthier. Pray about it because this is a needed change to your new lifestyle.

~Limit soda or diet drink intake. Work at making tea unsweetened or sweetened with non-calorie sweetener. You can also drink non-carbonated flavored waters. Coffee and hot teas are a great "go to" options but moderation is the key.

~Drink a cup of warm water with a fresh lemon squeezed into it every morning when you first get up. This helps me cleanse my liver naturally.

Drink plenty of water every day: Your body needs it! I focus on getting nutrients from my food and hydration from water.

~Add a multivitamin to your daily plan and (for women a 1200 mg calcium citrate supplement). I am not a big advocate of supplements but a good multivitamin is important for everyone!

~Eat 5 or 6 times a day: This is called stoking the fire. It keeps your metabolism working and fired up; working at burning those calories you are eating! Please remember to eat small meals. Focus on quality food in proper quantity.

~Eat all your vegetables, dairy and fruit servings allotted per day and pay attention to the "quantity" of food and the "quality" of the food you are consuming. No more skipping meals. You will actually slow your metabolism down by not eating breakfast and skipping meals.

~ Most Snacks should be between 100 and 200 calories. Choose fresh and healthy! Review the list of healthy snacks in chapter one.

~At the end of each day evaluate your day and make adjustments to the next day at the weakest point from the day before. Lose the mentality of giving up every time you get derailed in your program. Do the next right thing and remember this is a lifestyle change!

~Spread your calories around throughout your day. I think about it like this: I want to eat like a King at breakfast; a Queen at Lunch and a Pauper at my evening meal. I eat a blend of quality protein, complex carbohydrates and healthy fats at every meal throughout the day.

~Stock your pantry with healthy food. If it is in the pantry I will eat it and so will you. So clean out that pantry and make a commitment to yourself to refrain from bringing unhealthy food choices in the house. Ask family members to do the same. Enlist their help in making your home a haven of healthy food.

~Be careful about what you hear, see and believe. There is a lot of nutrition and diet information swirling around out there. Before you go and buy the latest greatest diet craze; gather the facts by looking for information published by registered dietitians, trained nutritionists, credible doctors and certified personal trainers. One of our FP4H Networking Leaders is a registered dietician; she has been a wealth of help and knowledge to me through my years of learning and also in teaching my FP4H classes. So find someone you can trust to help guide you. Then check it out before you buy it or try it!

~ If you are prone to hitting the drive-thru because you're pressed for time, you may want to consider preparing some healthy, easy-to-heat and eat meals ahead of time. You can prepare these and then re-heat when needed. This is a great way to cut down on the expense of eating out so much too.

With a little effort we can all take some baby steps to real change!

What in the World is Menu Planning?

Just what is menu planning? All it really means is that you "plan ahead of time" what meals you'll cook, prepare or even buy. Planning is an essential part of our everyday lives. Menu planning helps you stay on track with your new lifestyle; it saves hours of time, energy, money, and headaches, but it's easy to overcomplicate the process. And when that happens, it becomes a burden instead of a blessing. It is also a rewarding and effective way to track our calories. It does take time when we first start learning and planning. In no time at all you will be so much more organized and find that you are less prone to get off track.

Research has shown us that planning makes a difference in our weight loss efforts. By planning your menus; even when eating out you will avoid that last minute decision of what to eat, and where to eat; you will have it in your plan. You remove one more of the stumbling blocks on your journey to real and lasting success. It works but you have to work at it. Don't give up! And remember:
We will eat a meal whether we plan it or not. So plan!

I recommend menu planning at least a week at a time, and not going farther in advance than a month. Using this method I have enough menus planned to make it worth my while, yet not so scheduled that it becomes too big a chore. I want this to be as easy as possible. I use Google Calendar to plan my menus. I can streamline it with my Gmail account, so I can have it email me my day's menu and recipes each morning. I can plan a week's worth of simple dinners. Enter it on my google calendar so that it repeats two weeks later. I then plan another week of simple dinners. Enter it on the google calendar so that it repeats two weeks later. ~Walla – a month of dinners.

You can also go to: Google calendar menu planning and there will be tons of helps and guides that will come up that will help you navigate using Google to do all sorts of menu planning and meal preparation. It will take a little time in the beginning but after a few weeks it will get easier and easier to plan.

For those of us that are busier than ever and work outside the home you may want to invest in a program that you pay a nominal fee for that plans your menus and sends you the grocery list. I have never personally used them but have friends that love using this type program. Just check out google and see what you can find.

Other Helpful Information that has helped me in menu planning

~<u>Make a list</u> of the foods you love and plan them into your meal times. Remember this is not a diet but a new way of living. Some foods may need to be added daily, some only once a week and then some foods just need to be considered a once a month choice but build them into the plan and make it realistic for your lifestyle.

~<u>Try new dishes.</u> You might find that you family's taste will change, and adapt to new and healthier choices. Don't make the mistake of changing everything you are doing at once. It should be a slow process. Only one dish at a time can make the transition from unhealthy eating to healthy eating acceptable and positive for your family.

~<u>Check Out Restaurant menus online</u>. You will find that you make better food choices when you take the time to review the menu selection ahead of time. Make a list of acceptable restaurants and their healthy options and keep this list with you. Also don't be afraid to ask questions about food choices, ask   your servers for a to-go box ahead of time, ask the waiter/waitress to split your meal and only serve you half of it if this is possible.

~<u>Search for Resources.</u> Use the internet, my new cookbook; Simply Healthy Recipes, is a great "go to" resource, and any other recipe books that offer nutritional information on their recipes. Call your friends, take favorite family recipes and modify them to be healthy choices. You can replace ingredients that are reduced in fat, sodium and sugars and the flavor will not change in most cases. Use light or fat-free sour cream, salad dressing and mayonnaise when modifying recipes. Season your veggies with herbs, low fat ham, turkey or bacon. Small changes make a big difference. Try something new.

➤ Helpful websites I recommend for menu planning
There are many more to choose from. These are just some of the ones I use on a regular basis to help me in my meal planning efforts.

www.shopwell.com
www.dinnertool.com
www.livingrichlyonabudget.com/easy-menu-planning-ideas
www.livinglocurto.com/weekly-meal-plans
www.100daysofrealfood.com/our-free-meal-plans

I have included a complete chapter in this book on <u>Healthy Substitutions</u> as a resource. This will be a helpful "go to" guide for you as you begin to make needed changes to your recipes; so be sure to check them out in Chapter 5. This list is just some of the ones I use when I am creating new recipes or lovingly modifying some of my family's favorites.

Nutritional Information on Food Labels

~<u>Become a "Food Detective"</u> and learn the facts about the foods you are fueling your body with. Knowledge is powerful in the life change process. One of the websites that I love to use and that I recommend all the time to others is called Fooducate <u>www.fooducate.com</u>

This website helps me make healthier food choices all the time. So take time to check this one out. The Fooducate site rates the foods for you so it takes the guess work out of whether or not the food you have chosen is a healthy choice; Fooducate is available for iPhone, Android, and online so it is easy to use even while you are in the grocers.

Three other websites I use on a regular basis are:
www.firstplace4health.com
www.coachcalorie.com and
www.prayfit.com

All of these sites have good information. Please note I said "good" information. You have to determine what is right for you. My greatest help has come from being part of my FP4H group; it has given me accountability and strong group support which has really helped me stay on track with my health and fitness goals. First Place 4 Health has helped me find balance in all four areas of my life; mentally, emotionally, physically and spiritually. One of the best things you can do is to join a local FP4H group.

To search for a group near you go to the FP4H website and search for a group on the search function or get in touch with me at **glenna@netdoor.com** and I will help you find or start a group in your area.

My Nutrition Plan Cheat Sheet:

At times it is difficult to navigate the overwhelming amount of information available about a healthy eating. Remember this; focus on balance. Each person will need to personalize their food plan. Each of us is unique and all of us are very different. If this is going to be a successful "Lifestyle Change" then each person needs to invest some time into making this plan personal for them. An eating plan rich in a variety of nutrients from all the food groups will guide you to a healthy body. Here is a simple "cheat sheet" on the food groups that has helped me through the years to eating healthier.

~Fruits:
   ❖ Each serving of fruit normally contains 15 grams of carbohydrates, no protein, and no fat
   ❖ A serving is about a cup of fruit
   ❖ A cup serving of most fruit on average is about 60/70 calories per serving
   ❖ For the best nutritional value and fiber I use fresh or frozen fruit as much as possible
   ❖ In times when I use canned fruits I use only those packed in their own juice, pear juice or water
   ❖ If I have to use the fruit packed in syrup then I drain the syrup and rinse the fruit
   ❖ Most of us need about a cup and a half to 2 cups of fruit a day for a well balanced plan
   ❖ How many servings of fruit do you need a day? _____

~ Vegetables:
   ❖ Each serving of vegetables normally contains 5 grams of carbohydrates, 2 grams of protein and in most cases no fat
   ❖ A serving is about a cup of vegetables
   ❖ Except fresh leafy greens and the serving size is 2 cups

- ❖ Many vegetables contain about 25 to 30 calories for a cup serving
- ❖ The vegetables you should choose most often or fresh or frozen
- ❖ Starchy vegetables we should eat in moderation
- ❖ Beans are considered a vegetable and can be used as a meat source too
- ❖ Please remember to check the calories on the different types of vegetables you most often eat
- ❖ Most of us need about 2 to 3 cups of vegetables a day for a well balanced plan
- ❖ How many servings of vegetables do you need a day? _____

~Grains: (AKA: Bread/Starch)
- ❖ Each serving of grains normally contains 15 grams of carbohydrates, 3 grams of protein and a trace of fat
- ❖ A serving is 1 ounce of bread/grain
- ❖ Grains are normally about 70 to 80 calories for one ounce serving
- ❖ The grains you should choose most often should be whole grains
- ❖ Eat refined or processed grains in moderation
- ❖ Most of us need about 5 to 7 ounces of grains a day
- ❖ How many ounces of grains do you need a day? _____

~Milk/ Dairy Products:
- ❖ Each serving of Milk/Dairy normally contains 8 grams of carbohydrates, 12 grams of protein and the fat content is based upon the type of product you choose. Fat Free/trace of fat ~ Low Fat/3 to 5 grams of fat ~ Whole/8 grams of fat per serving. I choose the low fat varieties most often
- ❖ A serving is 1 cup for liquids and soft foods & 1 ounce for hard cheeses
- ❖ Milk/Dairy servings are normally about 80/90 calories for no fat ~ 105/120 calories for low fat and 150 calories for whole fat varieties
- ❖ Focus on calcium rich foods that are high in protein and low in sugar
- ❖ Most of us need 3 cups of Milk/Dairy a day for a well balanced plan
- ❖ How many cups of Milk/Dairy do you need a day? _____

~Meat (Protein)

- ❖ Each serving of Meat/Protein normally contains no Carbohydrates, 7 grams of protein and the fat content is based upon the type of product you choose. Lean/3 grams of fat ~ Medium Fat/5 grams of fat ~ High fat/8 grams of fat per serving. I choose the lean varieties as much as possible
- ❖ A serving size is 1 ounce
- ❖ Meat/Protein servings are normally about 55 calories for lean varieties ~ 75 calories for medium fat and 100 calories for high fat varieties
- ❖ Go lean with protein choose things with no legs which is fish or 2 legs which is chicken
- ❖ Most of us need 5 to 7 ounces of Meat/Protein a day
- ❖ How many ounces of Meat/Protein do you need a day? _____

~Healthy Oils

- ❖ Healthy Oils contain no carbohydrates, no protein and about 5 grams of fat per serving
- ❖ A serving size is 1 teaspoon
- ❖ Healthy Oils servings are normally about 45 calories each
- ❖ Focus on healthy oils which are unsaturated fats
- ❖ A relatively low fat eating plan if rich in variety will allow you enough of healthy fat without adding extras
- ❖ Most of us need 3 to 5 teaspoons of healthy oils a day
- ❖ How many teaspoons of Healthy Oils do you need a day? _____

Food Plan Objectives:

- ❖ Keep it simple
- ❖ Buy quality foods
- ❖ Eat in proper quantity
- ❖ Choose from all the food groups at every meal
- ❖ Moderation not depravation

My Nutrition Plan Changes:

Here is your opportunity to begin to build your plan. Think about it...then Take it to the next level! Write down some of your thoughts and changes you intend to make here.

What are some changes that I intend to make to my nutrition plan:

_____

_____

What are some items listed in this chapter that I am going to try:

_____

_____

 What other changes do I need to make?

_____

_____

Some websites I intend to look up and check out:

_____

_____

_____

Ways I intend to incorporate menu planning into my plan:

_____

_____

_____

All positive change starts with doing the next right thing. Just begin there and work your way toward a new way of life. Simple changes made today will impact your tomorrow.

Chapter 4 ~ My Top 12 Super Foods

What makes my super foods so super? My super foods all have something in common: They're all considered my favorites and they are all filled with nutrients that will help keep me healthy and feeling great from the inside out! Good nutrition starts here.

~<u>Blueberries</u>: Are high in antioxidants and have also been shown to help preserve memory function. Blueberries, like other berries, also have a high water content, which makes them hydrating for your skin and other cells of the body. I also use a blend of mixed berries; raspberries, blueberries, blackberries and strawberries. These berries are a great combo for smoothies and to top off yogurt.

~<u>Fish</u>: Is great because it provides a great source of essential fatty acids. Not only that, but it's high in DHA – an omega-3 fatty acid. Fish also contains plenty of lean protein for building fat-burning muscles. My top choices are salmon, rainbow trout and tuna.

~<u>Beans</u>: Are low in fat, high in fiber, high in protein, and very low on the glycemic index. Beans are a great source of protein. Being high in fiber and low on the GI scale, it provides a perfect metabolic environment for releasing and metabolizing fatty acids which is very important for fat burning. Black beans are my favorite.

~<u>Nuts</u>: Nuts are a great fat burning food. They are high in healthy fats, essential fatty acids, and fat soluble vitamins. They even have fiber and protein. The healthy fats you eat in nuts give a signal to your body that says "it's OK to release stored fatty acids because I'm providing you with plenty of them from my diet." This allows you to lose the fat and keep the muscle. Almonds and Pistachio nuts are my top picks.

~Eggs: Are a great fat-burning food in my opinion. We've been told over and over again that eggs are high in cholesterol and we shouldn't eat them. However, some recent studies show that dietary cholesterol has very little effect on blood cholesterol levels. Your body's cholesterol levels are typically a result of high arterial inflammation caused by processed carbohydrates. Free-range eggs are packed with essential fatty acids and protein – definitely a great combination for a fat-burning food. I usually eat egg beaters myself and try to have them every day with spinach, salmon and diced tomatoes. Please check with your doctor. Your super foods list may or may not need to include eggs.

~Broccoli: Is one of the highest sources of vitamin C. Many people associate vitamin C with fruit, but broccoli has 150% of the recommended daily allowance in just a single 100g serving. Broccoli is one of those foods that you can eat nearly an unlimited amount of and not have to worry about gaining weight. It's just too bulky and devoid of calories to overeat. This makes it one of my super foods. I love it steamed and also grilled.

~Spinach: Is filled with antioxidants, including vitamin C and beta-carotene, as well as lutein and zeaxanthin — a duo that acts like sunscreen for your eyes and guards against macular degeneration. One cup of fresh spinach leaves also provides almost double the daily requirement for vitamin K, which plays an important role in cardiovascular and bone health. Spinach is a great source of iron, which keeps your hair and nails strong and healthy. I use fresh spinach leaves in my smoothies, as a base for salads, on sandwiches or I sauté it and add to an omelet. I have a recipe in my cookbook for Warmed Spinach that is out of this world good. Check it out!

~ Oats: AKA Oatmeal: Whole grain oats are one of the best sources of soluble fiber, which, in addition to lowering cholesterol, helps keep blood sugar levels under control. A bowl of wholesome oats topped with berries and chopped nuts for extra nutrition make a great way to start your day. I sometimes add ½ cup of eggbeaters and a ½ cup of unsweetened almond milk to my oatmeal, microwave for a minute and a half and I have a great power food; Presto! Oatmeal Soufflé. It is like eating an oatmeal cookie for breakfast. It is fast, simple and oh so healthy.

~ **Sweet Potatoes:** Are a delicious member of the dark orange vegetable family, which lead the pack in vitamin A content. A baked sweet potato is also loaded with vitamin C, calcium, and potassium. It is truly one of my favorite super foods. You can also buy them in bulk and they last for a good amount of time in a cool dry place.

~ **Low fat or fat-free Plain Yogurt:** My favorite is the Dannon or Fage brands. Yogurt is higher in calcium than some other dairy products and contains a great source of other nutrients, including protein and potassium. It can also be enhanced with other good-for-you substances. Yogurt is a food that is rich with probiotics for a healthy balance of bacteria in your gut. It is also considered a heart healthy food. I also cook with yogurt. I use it in entrees, bakery items like cornbread and cakes, in dips for veggies and sauces. I sub it anywhere I would use milk or sour cream.

~**Quinoa:** Quinoa is a seed, not a grain and its grown high in the Andes Mountains of South America. Quinoa is stocked with nutrients all across the board, including all eight essential amino acids which make it a complete protein. There are other highly beneficial compounds, vitamins and minerals in quinoa. It is easy to prepare and can be added to many dishes. It takes on the flavor of the dish you add it to so it can be combined with so many things and taste great!
I make quinoa pancakes and I also add quinoa to soups, main dishes and even breakfast and snack foods. The possibilities are endless when it comes to using quinoa in your healthy food plan. Quinoa is pronounced ("keen-wah"). You can also find other food items like quinoa pasta and quinoa flour in the grocery shelves now. Try making the switch to some healthy quinoa products and make a change for the better.

~**Flax Seed Meal:** Ground flax seed is easier for your body to digest and whole flaxseed may pass through your intestine undigested, which means you won't get all the benefits if you take it in the whole state. So make sure you buy the ground flax seed meal or use a coffee grinder and grind your own.

Flax seed meal is high in fiber and omega-3 fatty acids, as well as phytochemicals called lignans. Flaxseed is commonly used to improve digestive health or relieve constipation. Flaxseed may also help lower total blood cholesterol and low-density lipoprotein (LDL, or "bad") cholesterol levels, which may help reduce the risk of heart disease. I add it to my yogurt, to smoothies, and when baking or grilling fish I sprinkle on a tablespoon or two of flax seed meal. I also add it to grilled tomatoes and it can also be used as an egg substitute in many recipes.

There you have it – my top 12 super foods. It's very simple to incorporate every single one of these into your healthy eating plan. Not only are they easy to incorporate, but they will help build the foundation for a healthy eating lifestyle that will be Life Changing for you! Now work on creating your list of Super Foods.

My Super Foods list will consist of:

_____

_____

_____

_____

_____

_____

_____

Prayer Journal:
At times in my journey there are foods that I have to really pray about adding to my plan. Maybe you have a food or two that you just need to pray about adding to your plan. A healthier choice that needs to be made....
Start with prayer:

_____

_____

_____

_____

_____

Chapter 5 ~ Healthy Substitutions

Here are some healthy substitutions that I use all the time. This is my personal list and I use them often when I am modifying recipes. I usually make the recipe up a few days in advance of the day I plan to serve it if it is the first time I have made the substitution, just in case I need to make some additional adjustments.

Instead of:	Use this:
Oil	Cooking sprays (like Pam) or nonstick pans (You're cutting the fat) 2/3 c. Unsweetened applesauce to replace 1 c. oil or butter (Gives good consistency without all the fat and can save over 100 calories) ½ applesauce & ½ buttermilk in equal amounts to equal the amount of vegetable oil, butter or margarine called for in recipe (Use a standard liquid measuring cup and add the applesauce with the liquid ingredients. Reduce the amount of added sugar if the applesauce is sweetened. Try not to over bake; low-fat recipes tend to dry out when over baked.)
Butter or margarine	Prune Puree (Replace butter with equal amount of prune puree and cut the calories in half, eliminate almost all of the fat and add a little fiber. Because of the color of the prunes, its best to use this swap in dark breads or brownies. The recipe will bake up denser and have more moisture.)

Butter or margarine (continued)	To make your own prune puree, blend 1 cup of pitted prunes with 6 Tablespoons hot water until smooth)
	Substitute Canola oil for up to half of butter in baked goods to reduce saturated fat
	1 c. of pureed beans, pumpkin or fruit to replace 1 c. of butter or oil
Shortening	Use Trans and Saturated Fat-free margarine (if you must!)
Flour (all purpose)	Whole-wheat flour for half of the called for flour in baked goods. (Whole-wheat flour is less dense and works well in softer products like cakes and muffins.)
	A can of Black beans, rinsed, drained and pureed can replace 1 cup of flour. (This swap cuts up to 200 calories and adds protein and is also gluten-free.
	Because of the color of the beans, its best for chocolate cakes or brownies.)
Cream	Fat-free half & half or evaporated skim milk (Using either of these swaps will remove some fat and calories while maintaining the consistency of your recipe.
	Pureed Sweet potato or pureed white potato (Replacing the cream with an equal amount of regular or sweet potato puree in a creamy soup can save you about 230 calories per ½ cup serving and it's a great dairy substitute for those lactose intolerant friends).
	Pureed carrots, mashed potato flakes or tofu.
Cream Cheese	Fat-free or low-fat versions of cream cheese or Fat-free Ricotta cheese or yogurt cheese (made from nonfat yogurt)

Milk	Fat-free (skim) or low-fat milk (Skim milk has more calcium and protein and less than 1 gram of fat, however making the switch can change the richness of your recipe).
Buttermilk	1 c. milk & 1 Tablespoon of lemon juice (Mix in small bowl and let stand for 5 minutes – saves you money and calories.) 1 c. plain yogurt to replace 1 c. buttermilk
Mayonnaise	Reduced-calorie and reduced-fat mayonnaise Greek yogurt in equal amounts to the mayonnaise (Even the light mayo still has over 3 times the calories and 11 times the fat of Greek yogurt – let's not even consider the full-fat version!)
Cheese	2% milk, low-fat or fat-free cheese (Choosing low-fat cheese will save you fat and cholesterol. Be sure to look for a low-fat cheese that's also low in sodium.)
Sugar	1 teaspoon of vanilla extract (Since we can't completely cut out all the sugar when baking, you can cut it in half and add 1 t. of vanilla extract for the same results. Assuming a recipe calls for 1 c. of sugar, this swap takes the sugar calorie count from 775 calories to about 400.) Splenda, Stevia or Replace 1 cup of sugar & substitute 2/3 c. Agave Nectar then reduce liquid in recipe by ¼ cup
Corn syrup	1 c. honey, maple syrup, rice syrup or agave nectar to replace 1 c. of corn syrup

Ground beef	Extra-lean or lean ground beef, ground chicken, ground turkey breast or meatless crumbles (Be sure to check the fat content on the packages.) (Still a good idea after browning the meat, to drain and rinse the fat.)
Lettuce, Iceberg	Arugula, chicory, collard greens, dandelion greens, kale, mustard greens, spinach, romaine, green leafy lettuce, spring mix (Whenever possible, replace iceberg lettuce with any other type of lettuce. Iceberg lettuce is mostly water content and has no nutritional value.)
Oil-based marinades	Balsamic vinegar, fruit juice or fat-free broth
Salad Dressings	Make your own! You control the fat, sodium and flavor. Search the internet for recipes and also check out the ones that are in my cookbook Simply Healthy Recipes. The Comeback Dressing is absolutely the best.
Pasta and rice (white)	Whole wheat pasta, brown rice, wild rice, bulgur. Whole wheat couscous and quinoa are great alternatives to pasta and rice, and much better for you.
Seasoning salt	Use fresh herbs, salt-free dried herb blends, garlic or fresh peppers
Milk Chocolate chunks	Use half the amount of mini milk chocolate chips or finely chopped dark chocolate (Using the mini chocolate chips still gives every bite the sweet flavor but by using less overall you cut the calories.

 If you sub dark chocolate you gain flavonoids that help keep blood vessels clear and flowing. |

My Nutrition Plan Changes:

Here is your opportunity to jot down your thoughts and ideas. Formulate some ideas for your new plan. Write down some of your thoughts and changes you intend to make here.

What are some changes that I intend to make to my nutrition plan:

_____

_____

_____

What are some of the substitutions listed in this chapter that I am going to try?

_____

_____

_____

What other changes do I need to make?

_____

_____

_____

What are some ideas not listed here that I want to try:

_____

_____

_____

Other thoughts or ideas:

_____

_____

_____

_____

For I know the plans I have for you," declares the LORD, "plans to prosper you and not to harm you, plans to give you hope and a future.
Jeremiah 29:11

What changes to my food plan must become a priority for me?

_____

_____

What have I learned so far that has impacted me the most?

_____

_____

Carole Lewis inspired me in her book *Hope 4 You* as she shared her story on how to walk with God, to work with God and to wait on God. Through my journey of weight loss and life change there are times that I must walk with God when I cannot see the plan, I must work with God as if the outcome depends on me and I must wait on God because his timing is perfect. My strength and ability really depends on him. Hope has been rekindled in my heart and God has done and is still doing a mighty work in me. Take a few minutes to reflect on the following places you might need to surrender to the Lord's plan for your life.

In what areas of my life do I need to <u>walk</u> with God?

_____

_____

In what areas of my life do I need to <u>work</u> with God?

_____

_____

In What areas of my life do I need to <u>wait</u> on God?

_____

_____

Chapter 6 ~ Setting Goals

Ever notice how we start well but have a hard time finishing?
Do you ever give much thought to this? What are some of the excuses you have used in the past about not finishing? Some of the reason's you don't finish?

Most of my excuses have been because I did not have a goal or a plan.

A goal is a "mark" on which to fix the eye. A goal should be a guiding positive force that motivates and encourages you.
A goal helps to evaluate or measure your efforts.
A Goal is a dream with a deadline:
It should give you focus and direction in each area of your life (that is why in FP4H we ask you to set goals in each area (mentally, emotionally, spiritually and physically)

I believe in setting goals (it keeps me going) I am going to share with you how I set goals and how you can be successful at doing it.

➤ **Long Term: Goals (you wish to achieve in the next 5 years) (this is my dream place) (I start with the End in Mind.)**
Why they are important: Goals help you anticipate success and change your life. Goals should always set us up for success not failure.

*<u>Physical</u>: How do I see my physical self changing in the next 5 years? (Run a full Marathon)
*<u>Mental</u>: (Example: get personal training license)
*<u>Emotional</u>: What would you like to change in your emotional makeup in the next 5 years? (Work on my anger)
*<u>Spiritual</u>: How would you like to grow in your Spiritual Life in the next 5 years? (Example: Memorize more scripture, revisit the Holy Land)

Develop at least 3 Long Term Goals

After setting my long term goals, the next step is to determine how you are going to achieve those goals. We do this by setting up some Short Term Goals.

➢ Short Term Goals (One Year Goals) these are goals that I will set to accomplish within the next year and these are goals that should help me accomplish my long term goals.

We all seem to fall into the trap of wishing but never doing.
Breaking down long term goals into short term goals will help us learn to follow through and chart our progress.
Writing down your goals will keep you accountable and can act as a reminder and motivator when you start to lose momentum.

Take each of your long term goals and set a one year goal that will move you toward achieving it:
Now take the next step which is to plan out a "90 day" game plan.
Now take the time to plan some "daily goals" which will help you put your plan into your schedule. This way we get to acknowledge our success everyday!

If you do not make "Life Change" a priority you will not reach your goals. You have to see yourself as important and valuable. Remember these tips:
    ➢ Set Realistic Goals (long term)
    ➢ Set Specific Goals (one year)
    ➢ Plan Ahead (90 days)
    ➢ Simple and achievable (Daily Goals) but be very specific

Last: Have a plan B (many of us get derailed because we have a plan and then it does not work out and we have no backup plan) Formulate Plan B....

Victory is not won in miles but in inches. Focus on the inch not the mile!

Further Goal Setting Tips

The following guidelines will help you to set effective, achievable goals:

➢ State each goal as a positive statement - Express your goals positively: "Execute this technique well" is a much better goal than "Don't make this stupid mistake."

➢ Be precise: Set precise goals, putting in dates, times and amounts so that you can measure achievement. If you do this, you'll know exactly when you have achieved the goal, and can take complete satisfaction from having achieved it.

➢ Set priorities - When you have several goals, give each a priority. This helps you to avoid feeling overwhelmed by having too many goals, and helps to direct your attention to the most important ones.

➢ Write goals down - This crystallizes them and gives them more force.

➢ Keep operational goals small - Keep the low-level goals that you're working towards small and achievable. If a goal is too large, then it can seem that you are not making progress towards it. Keeping goals small and incremental gives more opportunities for reward.

➢ Set performance goals, not outcome goals - You should take care to set goals over which you have as much control as possible. It can be quite dispiriting to fail to achieve a personal goal for reasons beyond your control!

➢ Set realistic goals - It's important to set goals that you can achieve. All sorts of people (for example, employers, parents, media, or society) can set unrealistic goals for you. They will often do this in ignorance of your own desires and ambitions. It's also possible to set goals that are too difficult because you might not appreciate either the obstacles in the way, or understand quite how much skill you need to develop to achieve a particular level of performance.

➢ Last thing-search the internet for free downloadable goal forms or just start with a journal or notebook and re-evaluate your goals often.

My Nutrition Plan Changes:

My Goal setting Plan to achieve my SMART Goals

Long Term Goals:

_____
_____
_____

Short Term Goals:

_____
_____
_____

Steps I am taking to accomplish my new goals:

_____
_____
_____

Daily Goals and the steps to achieve them:

_____
_____
_____

Ways I intend to incorporate goal setting into my plan:

_____
_____
_____

Additional thoughts or ideas:

_____
_____
_____

Chapter 7 ~ Your Metabolic Rate

What is basal metabolic rate? This is the number of calories your body burns at rest. It is based on things like age, height, and body type.

The metabolic rate can be influenced by numerous factors. We can change some of these factors, whilst others we have to accept. The most effective way of raising metabolic rate when trying to lose fat weight is to add more lean muscle to your body. Just an extra few pounds of muscle can boost the metabolism and help give you more shape.

Here are some factors that I have found Increase the Metabolic Rate:

Please note: there is a great deal of research being done on the metabolic rate and the internet is loaded with lots of information. You decide what is important for you.

- ➤ Body Size. A naturally big body means more cells to maintain which requires more calories; therefore larger people tend to have a high metabolism.
- ➤ Weight Gain. This speeds up the metabolism as each movement requires the contraction of more muscle to move the mass, even if the weight gained is fat. However fat is not metabolically active, so the metabolic rate will only be higher during movement.
- ➤ Body Composition. Body composition is the difference between total lean weight compared to fat weight. A higher percentage of lean body weight results in a high metabolic rate compared with individuals of the same weight with a higher fat percentage.
  A lean person burns many more calories than an overweight person at rest because lean body weight is metabolically active.
- ➤ Gender. Men naturally have a higher degree of lean muscle and research suggests this is mainly due to the male sex hormones resulting in the difference in body size and composition.

- Age. After 30 years of age there is usually a gradual decline in lean body weight and an increase in fat weight. This is mainly due to hormonal changes and will lead to a lowering of the metabolism. Regular exercise in adulthood will slow this process down and help keep metabolism up.
- Hereditary. Differences in genes can affect metabolism. Some people can have the same weight, fat content and age but have different body types which result in different metabolic rates. Other genes could influence fat uptake and utilization.
- Hormones. Hormones are chemical messengers that move through the bloodstream and control many of the body's main chemical processes and can so influence the metabolism. A rise in some of the body's important hormones through regular exercise can increase lean weight and change the body composition.
- Psychological State. Stress and anxiety can cause a rapid increase in energy expenditure. When a person is said to be "on edge" or nervous they are in a state of high alert, different hormones circulate the blood vessels and communicate to cells to break down energy stores ready to provide a greater supply of energy if needed.
- Temperature. If we are too cold we shiver which burns up much energy from the constant contraction and relaxation of muscle cells trying to produce heat to maintain a constant body temperature. When we are hot we also burn more calories through the process of sweating. When you train or exercise hard, at a fast pace, you are naturally increasing the temperature of your body.

The human metabolism is also affected by your eating habits. Overeating for example places a huge amount of stress on the hormones involved in metabolism. When you eat too much regularly, the excess food creates a hormonal imbalance which affects your energy levels and your ability to use calories efficiently. Eventually, this imbalance can lead to obesity, diabetes, cardiovascular disease and other serious health conditions.

Important Reasons to Increase Metabolism

An increased metabolism provides many benefits to help maintain continuous and permanent weight loss:

- Less exercise would be needed - giving you more time for other things
- Less effort if you did exercise - no need to try burning lots of calories during each session!
- Less chance of weight regain later
- Still enjoy some favorite foods – just learn to eat them in a healthier way
- Save money from not needing to buy junk food and other high calorie high fat foods
- Higher percentage of fat loss over fluid loss

Ways to Speed up the Metabolism

Want to keep your metabolism humming? I wanted to rev up my engine a little higher and keep my metabolism running. By making some simple adjustments to my plan this was possible and these tips will help you maximize your weight loss success as well:

- Strength Training: By strength-training just a couple of times a week I was able to increase my metabolism.

- Workout Intensity: I used a high intensity strategy for 30-second intervals, returning to my normal speed afterward.

- Eat More Fish: Omega-3s balance blood sugar and reduce inflammation, helping to regulate metabolism. I eat salmon about 3 times a week.

➤ <u>Build some Muscle</u>: Weight training twice a week will build muscle and reduce body fat. Building my muscle helped increase my resting heart rate and has helped re-set my metabolism.

➤ <u>Drink Green Tea</u>: Green tea has long been heralded for its antioxidant polyphenols. But new evidence shows the active ingredient, catechin, may crank up metabolism. I drink it every day!

➤ <u>Eat Often</u>: To keep that metabolism humming you need to eat small meals every three or four hours. I eat 5 to 6 meals a day.

➤ <u>Eat Enough Calories</u>: It's one of the most frustrating realities --if you cut out too many calories, your metabolism thinks times are lean and puts the breaks on fat-burning to conserve energy. Eat enough calories to at least match your resting metabolic rate.

➤ <u>Exercise</u>: Is a gift to yourself that keeps on giving. There is something out there known as excess post exercise oxygen consumption (EPOC), your body can take hours to recover from a robust workout (one intense enough that you can't hold a conversation) and return to its previous resting metabolic rate. The gift is your body is actually burning more calories than it normally would—even after you've finished exercising.

➤ <u>Eat Early</u>: Eating breakfast triggers a process called thermo genesis (this is the process where the body signals the brain to activate the metabolic process of turning food into energy. On the other hand not eating breakfast causes your brain to send a message to your cells to conserve energy (Your body then holds onto the fat stored in the cells instead of helping you burn it off); a nutrient-rich morning meal (like Oatmeal Soufflé or a spinach-and-salmon omelet with a slice of pita bread) shortly after getting out of bed literally wakes up your metabolism.

➢ <u>Eat more Protein</u>: Especially for breakfast! I spread my protein around during the day and make sure I have some protein at each meal and snacks if possible.

➢ <u>Sleep:</u> Last but not least get plenty of sleep. Sleep is intricately connected to various hormonal and metabolic processes in the body and is important in maintaining metabolic homeostasis. Research shows that sleep deprivation and sleep disorders may have profound metabolic and cardiovascular implications. Sleep is the best way for your body to rebuild.

Some "Fat Burning" Foods you need to have in your plan

~Wild Salmon	~Walnuts	~Eggs
~Quinoa	~Avocado	~Artichokes
~Lentils	~Coffee	~Blackberries
~Yogurt/Kefir	~Dark Leafy greens like kale & spinach	

There is so much information out on the web: Search out good information. Here are a few of the sites I use and recommend.

http://www.weightlossforall.com/factors-change-metabolism.htm
http://caloriecount.about.com/tools/calories-burned
http://caloriecount.about.com/tools/calories-goal

Questions I need to get answered:

Have I had a check up or complete physical in the last year?

_____

_____

Do I have any medical conditions that need to be resolved?

_____

_____

My Nutrition Plan Changes:

Write down some of your thoughts, ideas and changes you intend to make here.

What are some changes that I intend to make to my metabolic rate:

_____

_____

_____

What are some items listed in this chapter that I am going to try:

_____

_____

_____

What other changes do I need to make?

_____

_____

_____

Some websites I intend to look up and check out:

_____

_____

_____

Thoughts, ideas and plans:

_____

_____

_____

_____

_____

_____

Chapter 8 ~ Positive Affirmations

Positive Affirmations help us learn to change our thoughts on a daily basis. With affirmations from God's Word we can begin to change our hearts and minds and really being to see ourselves as God sees us. The key to the positive affirmations is to say them everyday ~ out loud. Yes I know how hard that is but you can do it.

I am beautiful, capable, and lovable.
I am valuable. I am precious to God.
I love myself unconditionally and nurture myself in every way.
I am special, unique and the apple of God's eye.

I am a beloved child of God.
I love people and show love, warmth, and friendship to all.
I am healed of all my childhood wounds, and I hold no account of wrong done to me. I am free from past hurts.
I can be honest with others and myself.
All of my relationships are based on integrity and respect.

I am intelligent and have great creativity.
I can concentrate and focus easily.
I can analyze and solve problems.
I learn quickly and have an excellent memory.
I have the mind of Christ.
I can make decisions with confidence.

I am diligent, faithful, and have a spirit of excellence.
Whatever I put my hand to will prosper.
God always causes me to triumph in Christ.
I let go of things I cannot control.
I have the courage to change the things I should change, the serenity to accept the things I cannot change, and the wisdom to know the difference.
I have no need to control people or situations.

I am controlled by the Holy Spirit.
I am a success and I trust God above all else.
I can do anything I put my mind to.
I can do all things through Christ, who strengthens me.
I see each day as a new and positive adventure.
I give thanks in all things and in all situations.

I express my potential more and more each day.
I see problems as exciting challenges that cause me to grow stronger and stronger in my faith.
I visualize myself as the person God wants me to be.
I see myself achieving my goals and fulfilling God's purpose for my life.

I live every day with passion and power.
I feel strong, excited, passionate, and powerful.
I feel tremendous confidence and self worth because of Christ.
I have all the abilities I need to succeed in Christ.

Every cell in my body vibrates with health, healing, vitality, and love.
I am healthy and strong and filled with vitality.
Jesus took every sickness and every disease away from me.

I awaken each day feeling healthy and alive with energy.
Any tension I feel is simply a signal to relax, release, and let go.
I always have more than enough energy to do all I want to do.

All that I am, I derive from Jesus.
He is always in my thoughts, and I pray without ceasing.
Jesus is my strength, my joy, my peace.
He is with me wherever I go, and He promised never to leave me or forsake me.
I am free, happy and healed in the name of Jesus.

Chapter 9 ~ Progress Check–Up

I felt it was important to add this chapter for several reasons. The first one being that to really decide where we need to go or be we need to evaluate where we are. Each year at least twice a year I do a progress check up. It helps me re-focus on my plans and goals. It also helps me realize what I have not accomplished. You are not turning this in to anyone. Be honest with yourself so you can continue to improve and take the best care possible of your body. Consider this a quiz that you get to grade…..

1. **Am I eating within my calorie range every day? This means not below or above.**   O Yes   O No   O Sometimes

2. **Am I exercising at least 3 times a week for at least 45 minutes?**
    O Yes   O No   O Sometimes

3. **Am I doing some type of Bible reading or Bible study daily?**
    O Yes   O No   O Sometimes

4. **This past week did I eat 3 meals a day?**   O Yes O No

5. **This past week did I have 2 or 3 <u>healthy</u> snacks each day?** O Yes   O No

6. **Did I have 2 or 3 dairy products each day?** O Yes   O No

7. **Did I have at least 2 to 3 cups of vegetables each day?** O Yes   O No

8. **Were most of the vegetables I ate this week fresh and or frozen?**
    O Yes   O No   O Sometimes

9. **Were most of my vegetables non starchy?** O Yes   O No

10. Did I eat 2 or 3 pieces of fruit a day?   O Yes   O No

11. Were half of the grains I ate each day whole grains?   O Yes   O No

12. Did I limit my grains to the proper number of ounces for me? O Yes   O No

13. Did I limit my meat to the proper number of ounces for me? O Yes   O No

14. Am I eating lean meats?   O Yes   O No   O Sometimes

15. Have I quit eating fried foods? O   Yes   O No   O Most of the times

16. Am I still eating foods that only have empty calories on a daily basis? (No value to the body or for the body is empty calorie foods)
    O Yes   O No   O Sometimes

17. Am I reading the nutritional labels on the foods I am considering purchasing so I can make good choices?   O Yes   O No   O Sometimes

18. Do I pray about what I am going to eat? O Yes   O No   O Sometimes

19. Am I planning my meals ahead of time? O Yes O No O Sometimes

20. Am I thankful that I can choose to eat healthy foods and am I demonstrating a positive attitude?   O Yes   O No   O Sometimes

21. Am I mad and or bitter that I can't eat the things that I think I want even though it is harmful to my body?   O Yes   O No   O Sometimes

22. Am I tracking my food each day? O Yes   O No   O Sometimes

23. Have I set some long term goals for my Life Change plan?
    O Yes   O No

24. Have I created a backup plan for myself so when things don't go as planned I have another resource to fall back on? O Yes   O No

25. Do I have an accountability partner that I can trust?
     O Yes   O No   O Sometimes

I pray that this quiz will be helpful to you so that you will truly learn to take good care of this temple that Almighty God has given you to live in. Good Health is about finding balance in your life. It's about the hope, joy, peace and strength we find in all 4 areas of our lives when we focus on being balanced; mentally, physically, spiritually and emotionally. It is about being all Christ wants us to be in Him. Remember He is LIFE!

"Do you not know that your bodies are temples of the Holy Spirit, who is in you, whom you have received from God? You are not your own; you were bought at a price. Therefore honor God with your bodies." I Cor. 6: 19-20

My Nutrition Plan Changes:

Write down some of your thoughts and changes you intend to make:

_____
_____
_____
_____
_____
_____
_____
_____
_____
_____

A Matter of Prayer ~ A New Life demands a New Lifestyle

Jesus said to her, "I am the resurrection and the life; he who believes
in Me will live even if he dies, and everyone who lives and believes
in Me will never die. Do you believe this
John 11:25-26

Food For Thought:

Jesus has power over life and death as well as power to forgive sins. Whoever
believes in Christ has a spiritual life that death cannot conquer. This is because
He is the Creator of Life! When we realize His power and how wonderful his
offer to us really is it should empower us to commit our lives to Him. It should
empower us to make a real lifestyle change, not temporary improvement but
real change!

When we allow God to work in us we begin to hear his promise of freedom.
Remember He is the creator of life! God focuses on the "total person" and He
wants to touch our life in all areas: the physical, mental, emotional and the
spiritual. When we allow Christ to speak into our life just like Lazarus we will
hear Christ speak freedom to us. Lazarus heard the Father's voice and he chose
to come forth from the tomb and we can too! Do you hear the promise of
freedom! Christ is calling you!

Action Step:
We cannot continue to keep doing the same things we have been doing and
expect different results. Begin today to develop a plan for change.

Prayer for Today:
*Lord, I know that the Life I have been living is not the one you would choose for
me. You have a life of true abundance for me. Empower me today to see the truth
of your word. Touch me in the deepest place of my need and begin your healing
work that only can be accomplished through the power of the Cross. Help me to
begin to make healthy choices that truly will be life changing!*

Chapter 10 ~ Exercise Tips

The only real requirement is to start and remember you deserve to give yourself time to exercise, we are better at the other things we have to do if we take time to exercise. We are more balanced with our whole plan if we include exercise in our plan. So plan that exercise!

Make this an appointment on your calendar. Do something! When exercising at the right level of effort the body, mind and spirit come together to produce a feeling of great satisfaction.

Exercise can be and is restorative and refreshing. The stress release from exercise is almost immediate and empowering!

The real key is to have patience and don't give up! Have fun and enjoy the journey.

Here are some Exercise Tips that helped me get started:

➢ Just 10 minute segments of exercise throughout your day COUNT. This has really helped me and will help anyone; especially those that have long work days. American Heart says 3-4 (10minute) work outs throughout your day are great. It really helped me when longer workouts used to really scare me. Let's face it the bigger you are the harder it is to stay at it or to even get started; so break it up and do something! I didn't want to think about doing anything for 30 minutes or an hour, but 10 minutes was doable!!!

➢ Mix it up. Be sure and cross – train. Every little bit counts! Try to change up your daily workout. If you miss your daily work out; you can still fit something in. Watch one of your favorite TV shows and do strength training moves during the commercial breaks: lunges, squats, and crunches. Remember mix it up. Giving yourself mini, achievable health goals can go a long way. Mix it up in whatever you do. Fun is the key to continuing!

➢ Change up your scenery. Workouts can get a little boring so trade the treadmill for some new terrain and explore a great path in your neighborhood. Go for a long hike or a swim. A new environment can breathe some fresh air into your routine and it also keeps your body guessing. So can trying different activities if you are a "gym junkie," then simply try different machines or weights, but keep it interesting.

➢ Do not use food as a reward. Rewards are very important when it comes to an exercise program and in some cases they can be crucial. Provide rewards that will keep you motivated and on track to your goals. New shoes or clothes, a massage, a special trip to an event that you want to go to are all great suggestions that work.

➢ Leave that magazine at the house. It might seem like a great way to keep yourself entertained during a workout but the truth is if you can read captions in a magazine, chances are you're not pushing yourself hard enough. If you're really feel a need to read then try downloading a podcast or listening to an audio book but the key is to make that workout count!

➢ Buddy up. All I can say is I could not make it without my buddies. Working out with a friend is a great way to stick with a fitness routine. Meet each other for a run in the morning or take an aerobics class before or after work. Just make sure you partner up with a pal you can count on to push you and help you reach your goals not one that will be your partner in the crime of not following through!

➢ Changing it up gets that metabolism going! Change up your workouts with a little high-intensity strength training. Increase the weight, reps and/or sets you lift (and decrease the amount you rest in between) and you'll start to see some sculpted, lean muscles (and you'll keep your metabolism humming post-workout!) Also break it up. Break up the monotony by putting a set of abs in between each set of your weight-training routine. Since you never have a chance to sit still and cool off, you'll keep your heart rate up and burn more calories and body fat. That is the key to a great workout!

➢ It is important to dress for success. Comfort above all else counts when it comes to shoes and clothes for exercising. Before you start any kind of exercise routine make sure that your body is well supported. This means comfortable shoes that are a good quality, if you are a woman; a strong support sports bra (or two) and high quality and very supportive underwear, breathable fabrics in shorts and shirts. You can focus on achieving better results instead of uncomfortable fitting clothing if good choices are made ahead of time. Remember to be successful at real life change we must have the right tools. I use to say the right clothes and underclothes keep the flip flop in place!

➢ Another great tool for exercise is a good step counter and or a heart rate monitor. I never exercise without my polar heart rate monitor; it keeps track of every calorie burned.

➢ Music has an amazing power to pump us up and get us going. Rather than relying on others to get you through a workout at times; try to organize some high energy and up-lifting songs on an I-pod or MP3 player. Put your favorite songs at the beginning, middle and toward the end of the time you'll be working out to motivate you. Change it up every week by adding new songs or switching Mp3 players with a friend. Music is a great motivator for all of us.

➢ Have some patience! It took years to accumulate fat and it is really best to burn it off gradually. The key is to keep it off forever from this point on. The goal is to establish a positive relationship with exercise. We want to learn to LOVE exercise!

➢ Chaffing Issues: During warm weather for most of us and for larger people that exercise regularly this can be a problem. We have areas where clothing or body parts produce wear on other body parts.

Reducing the friction in those areas will reduce the irritation. You can reduce friction and aggravation by using Vaseline and exercise products like "body glide". Compression tights (these are shorts made of Lycra) have reduced chaffing between the legs dramatically. I still wear compression shorts to workout in; it just makes good sense to me.

➢ Excess skin: Use compression tights, girdles, spandex, or they make a knee to chest undergarment that is like a panty but much more supportive which are designed for men and women. These types of undergarments help keep the excess skin from getting in the way. Also make sure you dry off properly and shower right after every workout, walk or run. Excess skin and moisture are a prime habitat for ulcers, skin rashes and yeast infections.

➢ Set doable short term goals for yourself. Once you reach that goal immediately set another one. Also helping others train for a goal is so motivating; this way you can help others while still helping yourself!

➢ Don't quit! Never give up on yourself. Exercise is the key to creating your fat burning furnace. Remember do something every day. Exercise will make you feel better and is a critical component to the life change process. If you fall of the wagon; just dust yourself off and start over. It is only failure if you don't get back up!

➢ Let's Move……..Here is a chart of some of my favorite activities. The activities listed below are showing calories burned per hour (energy expended) for a 130, 155, 180 or 205 pound person. The amount of calories expended is influenced by many factors, including body weight, intensity of activity, conditioning level and metabolism. I want to stress again these are suggestions; you must invest some time into creating your own list. There are many apps and different types of fitness equipment on the market today that will track your numbers for you on a more accurate level.

I wear a Polar FT60 that monitors my heart rate when I work out. You decide what is best for you. Develop a plan that fits......

Activity (1 hour)	130 lb	155 lb	180 lb	205 lb
Aerobics, general	384	457	531	605
Cycling, <10 mph, leisure bicycling	236	281	327	372
Cycling, 12-13.9 mph, moderate	472	563	654	745
Cycling , stationary bike moderate	413	493	572	651
Dancing, general	354	422	490	558
Dancing, slow ballroom	177	211	245	279
Health club exercising	325	387	449	512
Pushing a wheelchair	236	281	327	372
Running, general	472	563	654	745
Stretching, mild	148	176	204	233
Swimming, treading water, fast, vigorous	590	704	817	931
Swimming, treading water, moderate	236	281	327	372
Spin, biking class at the gym	426	487	578	623
Walking the dog	177	211	245	279
Walking 3.5 mph, brisk pace	354	422	490	558
Walking 4.0 mph, very brisk	295	352	409	465
Walking 4.5 mph	372	443	515	586
Walking 5.0 mph	472	563	654	745
Water aerobics, water calisthenics	236	281	327	372
Weight lifting, light workout	177	211	245	279

Exercise was and still is a critical component to my "life Change" process. I urge you to seek medical advice and get a wellness work up before starting any exercise program. Always be willing to seek out professional help. Adults that exercise are positive role models and get this; mothers who exercise are the most powerful role models to their own children. So lead by example.

We need to be positive role models spiritually, physically, mentally and emotionally for our children and others. Healthier kids become happier kids what a great combination and this fact alone should motivate us to learn to love exercise and pass it on!

What is stopping you? Whatever it is, it is time to let it go, move forward and see the truth and power in exercise. No more excuses! The evidence is growing that exercise will bring quality and longevity to your life and relationships. It will also bring to you better health; mentally, emotionally, physically and spiritually! It is really "Life Changing"! I'll see you at the finish line!

My Nutrition Plan Changes:

Write down some of your thoughts and changes you intend to make here.

What are some changes that I intend to make to my exercise plan:

_____

_____

_____

_____

What are some exercise tips listed in this chapter that I am going to try?

_____

_____

_____

What is one new thing I am going to try this week?

_____

_____

_____

What is one benefit of adding exercise to my plan?

_____

_____

Chapter 11 ~ Grocery Shopping Tips & Tools

Good nutrition starts with smart choices in the grocery store. Cooking up healthy meals is a challenge if you don't have the right ingredients in your kitchen.

But who has time to read all the food labels and figure out which items are the most nutritious and the best buys? Grocery shopping can be a daunting task, simply because there are so many choices.

This handy guide would not be complete without a few tips on grocery shopping and a copy of my own personal grocery list must haves for you. I have a grocery list on my computer that I use weekly that I created from a list on the shop well website. Glenn and I keep the grocery list on the kitchen counter and when we run out of something it goes on the list. If it is not on the list we don't buy it. Just one of the ways we prevent unhealthy foods from entering the house.

Here are some other great shopping tips that help me:

➢ Shop the perimeter of the grocery store, where fresh foods like fruits, vegetables, dairy, meat, and fish are usually located. Avoid the center aisles where junk foods lurk.

➢ Choose "real" foods, such as 100% fruit juice or 100% whole-grain items with as little processing and as few additives as possible. If you want more salt or sugar, add it yourself.

➢ Stay clear of foods with cartoons on the label that are targeted to children. If you don't want your kids eating junk foods, don't have them in the house.

➢ Avoiding foods that contain more than five ingredients, artificial ingredients, or ingredients you can't pronounce.

➢ Eat and buy a variety of nutrient-rich foods. You need more than 40 different nutrients that I know of for good health, and no single food supplies them all. Your daily food selection should include bread and other whole-grain products; fruits; vegetables; dairy products; and meat, poultry, fish and other protein foods. How much you should eat depends on your calorie needs.

➢ Eat before you go grocery shopping. Skipping meals can lead to out-of-control hunger, often resulting in overeating and over buying. When you're very hungry, it's also tempting to forget about good nutrition.

➢ Chocolate Peanut Butter: Is one of the best things that ever happened to me! It makes a great pre-work out snack, is good at breakfast, snack, lunch or dinner. It is a high quality food and gives me that little chocolate fix without empty calories or bad fats.

➢ Hummus is another great food I have discovered along the way in this journey. There are lots of great varieties out there. It can be used by itself or in combination with a small amount of salsa to create a spread for sandwiches, a base for dips, and can be added to chicken or turkey salad. It can take the place of mayonnaise in many different ways.

Following is a list of food items that are on my grocery list:

<u>Dairy section</u>
*Plain Greek yogurt- non fat
*Eggs
*Egg Beaters
*Low fat or no fat cottage cheese
*2% sharp cheddar cheese
*Hummus

Meats (you can freeze these if you buy in bulk)
*Chicken breasts
*Turkey breasts
*Lean beef
*Sirloin steak
*Fish (tilapia, salmon, cod, shrimp, mahi mahi)-any of these are good choices
*Tuna or Salmon or Turkey in a can or pouch packed in water

Fruits/Veggies
*Fruits (blueberries, strawberries, pineapple)
*Dried or frozen beans
*Mixed frozen vegetables (not in a sauce) Birdseye has some great mixes of
  fresh veggies like broccoli, baby carrots, water chestnuts and edamame beans
*Leafy greens ~ spring mix ~kale ~ leaf lettuce ~ romaine or swiss chard
*Spinach (I buy fresh and then freeze)
*Sweet potatoes
*Dry beans

Seasonings
*Lemon & pepper
*Garlic powder
*Mrs. Dash
*Ginger
*Turmeric
*Cayenne pepper
*Chili powder
*Coriander
*Fresh herbs (some of these I actually grow in my back yard in a flower pot and
      as they mature I will break them off and crush the leaves and put them in
      a zip lock container in the freezer.)
      Then when I need fresh herbs they are always on hand.

Other Food Items

*Flax seed meal (ground)

*Plain oatmeal (1 minute Quaker oats)

*Whey Protein powder (vanilla) I can get this at Sam's but I prefer buying online from allstarhealth.com because it is cheaper. I use this in my smoothies.

*Peanut butter all natural
 make sure it has no Hydrogenated Vegetable Oil in it

*Chocolate peanut butter (Sweet Dreams is the brand I buy)

*Brown rice cakes (Suzie's is the brand I use)

*Brown rice (Uncle Ben's)

*Joseph's bread (Pita) for wraps and pizza

*7 grain sprouted gluten free raisin bread in the freezer section because it has no preservatives in it. It is considered a health food so you will find it in the health food section of most grocery stores.

*No calorie Vitamin Water (many flavors to choose from)

*Plain bottled water

*Green tea (I drink the Lipton diet green tea with citrus or berry flavor)

Please note: This is not an exhaustive list but just some simple helpful tips I have learned along the way in my own personal journey. I have learned that there is no good or bad food. All food is permissible for me but not all food should have a prominent place in my food plan. The best place to begin is to make a list of the foods you really like and figure out a way to put them in your plan.

Moderation not deprivation is the real "Key" to success!

I have other additional tips and recipes in my new cookbook. *Healthy Living Made Simple ~ Food for the Body and Soul*. You can purchase a copy on Amazon.com or you can just e-mail me at glenna@netdoor.com and I will be happy to mail a copy to you.

Cooking healthy and light is easier than you think and it is Oh so delicious!

My Nutrition Plan Changes: Creating a Grocery List

Are you ready to take it to the next level..... Write down some of your thoughts and changes you intend to make here.

What are some changes that I intend to make to my grocery shopping:

_____
_____
_____

What are some items listed in this chapter that I need to add to my list:

_____
_____
_____

What other changes do I need to make?

_____
_____
_____

Some websites I intend to look up and check out:

_____
_____
_____

Additional thoughts and ideas:

_____
_____
_____

Grocery List:

Fresh Fruits:

_____

_____

_____

_____

_____

_____

Vegetables:

_____

_____

_____

_____

Dairy Section:

_____

_____

_____

_____

Meats:

_____

_____

_____

_____

Grains:

_____

_____

Seasonings:

_____

_____

_____

Special Food Items:

_____

_____

_____

_____

Other Food Items:

_____

_____

_____

_____

_____

_____

_____

_____

_____

Grocery Store Notes:

_____

_____

_____

Chapter 12 ~ Helpful Resources

I am a firm believer in getting all the help I can. That is the reason I wanted to add this resource page to the book. All of these resources and websites are useful tools. Plain and simple they will not take the place of your hard work and diligence but they can make the journey easier to travel!

Resources: These resources have helped me and will enhance your journey to good health.

~Portion Control Plate: One of the best tools ever created! I have seen great success with this helpful tool. It really helps get our portions under control. The key is to use it! Studies show people who use the plate method not only lose weight but learn to keep it off because they learn the value of portion control. It can be used at work~ home ~ or even in a restaurant. This plate is helpful with children and adults.
This particular one is designed to aid you in getting your portions correct on whatever you eat until you get a good understanding of a well balanced food plan. It is a great starting place and it really helped me finish the race! It comes with directions on the plate method of use and how to balance out your meals as well as a sample day of meals and some other helpful suggestions for your new lifestyle!
Can be ordered at: glenna@netdoor.com or www.joyceainsworth.com

~Food Scales: these are a great resource to help you get on track and stay on track. I weigh and measure my food. Even if you are on maintenance you need to continue to measure and weigh your food. Invest in a good quality scale; it will be well worth the investment. There are several out there that are good quality and easy to use. Email me for more info on this.

~Strength and Flexibility Bands: I love the variety of exercise I can do with these! They are great for travel, work, gym or home fitness plans. Fitness bands are available in many variations. I recommend bands that can work every major muscle group in the body. Strength and flexibility bands are a great addition to any workout plan. Spend some time and figure out how you fit these into your workout regimen. Fitness bands can be purchased at most fitness stores like Academy Sports or Dicks Sporting Goods. They can also be ordered at: Amazon.com or check out the selection offered at www.firstplace4health.com

~Other helpful tools for this new lifestyle can be found and ordered at www.firstplace4health.com They offer many resources that will help you become successful healthy living and more balanced in all areas: mentally, emotionally, physically and spiritually! Check out the website and sign up for the e-newsletter that they send out once a month. They offer a wealth of help and information through the e-newsletter and it is free; all you need to do is sign up. What a great way to be encouraged and inspired!

Helpful Websites for Success

➢ For all types of information and resources @ www.firstplace4health.com
➢ Healthy weight calculator @ www.cdc.gov/healthyweight/assessing/bmi
➢ Center for Disease Control @ www.CDC.gov
➢ 2010 Dietary Guidelines: @ www.DietaryGuidelines.gov
➢ A government web site where you will find information and tools to help you and those you care about stay healthy: @ www.healthfinder.gov
➢ Physical Activity Guidelines: @ http://www.health.gov/paguidelines
➢ Portion Distortion Quiz: National Heart, Lung, and Blood Institute Obesity Education Initiative @ http://www.nhlbi.nih.gov/about/oei/index.htm
➢ Healthy eating on a budget: @ www.choosemyplate.gov/healthy-eating-on-budget.html
➢ Online food and activity trackers can be found at the following sites: @ www.myfitnesspal.com, @ www.mypyramidtracker.gov, @ www.livestrong.com, @ www.calorieking.com
➢ Kids: @ http://teamnutrition.usda.gov/resources/mpk_worksheet.pdf
➢ National Christian weight loss program @ www.firstplace4health.com

About the Author

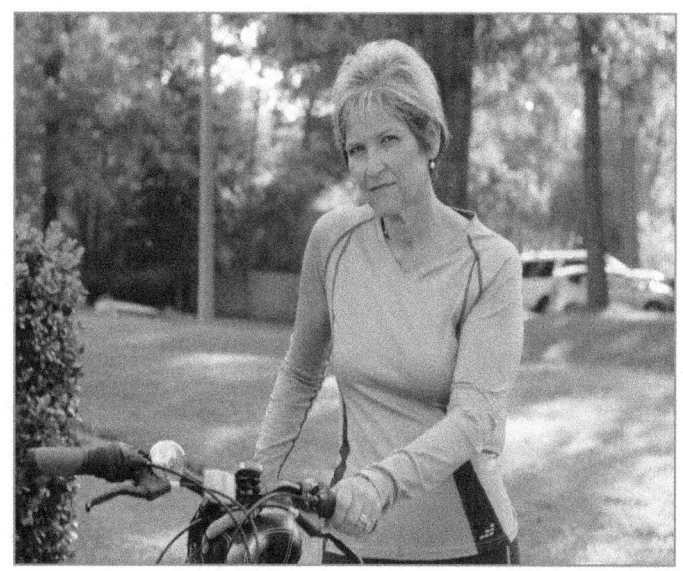

Joyce Ainsworth has been a lifetime resident of Mississippi, a dedicated wife to husband Glenn and mother to their five children; now grown. Through FP4H, she has been successful at losing and maintaining a weight loss of 192 pounds. Joyce speaks at seminars, conferences, and other events throughout the country. She coordinates the FP4H Ministry for her home church and teaches FP4H classes. She also serves as Regional Team Leader for FP4H for the Southern States of the United States.

As a successful business owner turned author and motivational speaker, she shares her experiences, offers insight, and is committed to helping others find hope, help, and healing out of the bondage to food and other addictions. Joyce is a member of the AWSA (Advanced Writers and Speakers Association), she is also a ISSA Certified Specialist in Fitness Nutrition and conducts cooking demonstrations and workshops on healthy living for a better life.

"Freedom is not a program," she says, "It is a lifestyle."

Her Motto:
Change Your Mind~ Change Your Body~ Change your Life!

Invite Joyce Ainsworth to speak at your next event

Contact her for a list of speaking topics
Email: glenna@netdoor.com   or   www.joyceainsworth.com

Read Joyce's weekly blog
Mondaymotivationsbyjoyce

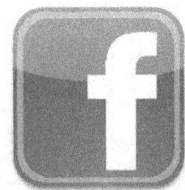

Connect with Joyce
Facebook – Joyce Ainsworth

@joyceainsworth

Read more about Joyce at:
http://www.firstplace4health.com/stories/34/joyce_ainsworth

Joyce's new Cookbook is now available:
Simply Healthy Recipes ~ Food for the Body and Soul
Taste and See How "Good" healthy can be!

Order your copy today at glenna@netdoor.com
Or at www.joyceainsworth.com
Copies are also available on Amazon.com

New Book Coming in Fall of 2015:
Healthy Living Made Simple
Changing your Mind & Loving your Body

WHAT FOLKS ARE SAYING ABOUT
FOOD FREEDOM AND FINISH LINES

Joyce has written a book that is going to encourage you to do the hard work of change—change that will last a lifetime. I love Joyce and believe that she has discovered the secret to losing weight and keeping it off. God's love language is obedience and when we do His work, His way, we will succeed. You are going to love this book as much as I do!
--- Carole Lewis, National Director, First Place 4 Health

Food, Freedom and Finish Lines will tell you how to be a big loser!! Here you will discover the incredible story of how Joyce Ainsworth lost 192 pounds. I love this book because it is so real and practical. Every page contains helpful tips on living a healthy lifestyle. Read and apply it now to make the most of the rest of your life.
---Steve Reynolds, Pastor, Capital Baptist Church, Annandale, VA., Author of
Bod4God and *Get Off The Couch*

FIVE STAR REVIEWS FROM AMAZON

One of the best books I have ever read. Truly life changing, and all the glory is given to the Lord by the author. An incredible story and I love the way she relates her journey to running. Look for this book to be a "best seller." Start your life change today—read the book! ---Donna

Joyce Ainsworth shares some very painful parts of her life in this revealing book, as an inspiration for others to understand that losing weight must begin on the inside. She helps the reader face reality about how they arrived at their current weight. She gives practical-no-bones ideas about the how-to of making lifestyle changes that are doable. She doesn't just tell how she lost over 192 pounds; she makes it visibly possible for the reader to believe that it is also possible for them. Joyce is a motivating speaker who is real and her compassion for others is real. This book hopefully, is just the first of her victory story! ---June

Finally! I've been "trying" to lose weight for over 30 years! This book finally told me how with no punches pulled. Nothing "warm and fuzzy" about this lady. LOL I weigh less now than I have in 25 years and have run two 1/2 marathons. Thank you Joyce.   ---Dave

To order your copy of:
>Food, Freedom and Finish Lines!
>>How to Lose the Weight and Win Back Your Life

Call today: 601-927-8974 or email me @ glenna@netdoor.com